The Modern Woman's Guide For A Stress Free Lifestyle

by Stacy Shakespeare

All Rights Reserved. No part of this publication may be reproduced in any form or by any means, including scanning, photocopying, or otherwise without prior written permission of the copyright holder. Copyright © 2016

Table of Contents

1. The Modern Day Working Family Woman
2. The Stress Response
3. Sources of Stress
4. Learn and Recognize the Signs of Stress
5. Techniques for Confronting and Managing Stress
6. Conclusion
7. THANK YOU FOR READING!

1. The Modern Day Working Family Woman

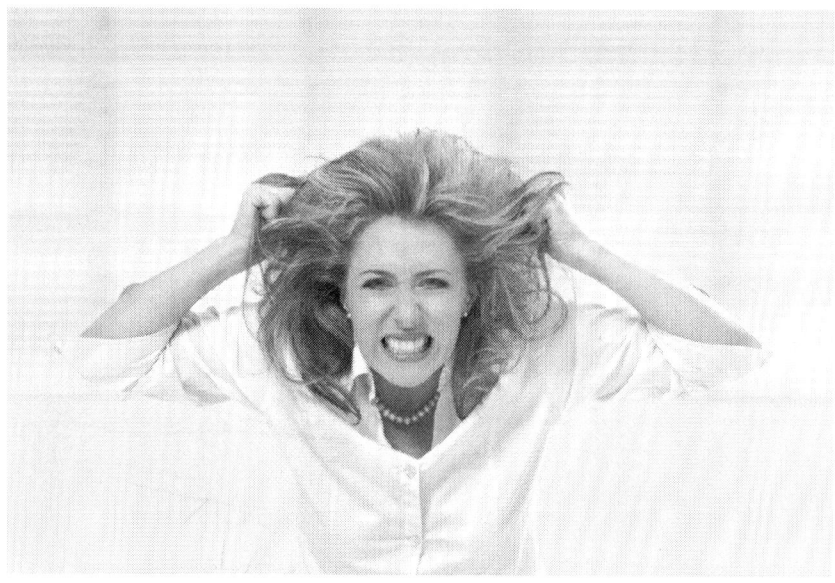

Women have a new role in current times, one which has shifted from the days of the past. Women have fought for equal rights, for the right to vote, for our place in the corporate ladder; but what is the cost? The answer seems to be stress. From a themed Thomas the Train party for your baby's first birthday, to presenting a new product in a board meeting, and don't forget having a delicious dinner on the table 15 minutes after you walk in the door; a professional family woman has her work cut out for her. Not to say that it is not possible, but it is a challenge which requires great effort, a strategy and techniques to balance the many roles. This is the challenge of the modern woman.

I have experienced life in a demanding work environment and can relate on many levels. Ten years ago now, I graduated from college and was set on a path to a successful career in the male-dominated corporate world. I wanted to make a successful life for myself and had the skills to do so. I dreamt of all the things I would be able to achieve. Of course, along with goals of achievement, came dreams of my life with my fiancé. We were engaged and planned to raise a family together. We set our minds on what we wanted to do, which was balance our work with our family.

Soon after I graduated from college, I was married and continued to climb the corporate ladder. I enjoyed my career, it challenged me and gave me purpose, but I also wanted to start a family. I prepared for challenges involved with balancing a family and a career by planning how I could manage my work hours, day care and free time. I worked it all out. However, I have learned some things just can't be planned for. I had no idea about the amount of stress I would face in my daily life. I didn't know the feeling I would experience when I get a call that my child is sick at daycare. Work matters just have to take the back seat. Late sleepless nights combined with early morning alarm clocks often left me completely exhausted. It was a struggle to balance my priorities between my husband, child and professional career. Spit up doesn't go well with a black suit.

While my story may seem difficult, I know I am not alone. Many women face lives full of stress and exhaustion. A lot is expected from a woman that balances a career and family life, and it can be tough, to say the least.

It is estimated that the amount of women who work to support their families rose from 38 percent in 1988, to 47 percent in 2009. This increase in workload for women, contributes to an increasing amount of stress. Women report being more stressed than men as a whole. In fact, on a scale from 1-10, 23 percent of women would rate their level of stress as an 8-10. The average woman's stress is 5.3 while the average men's stress level is 4.6.

Stress and Health

The problem with stress is that it has more of an effect on a women's life than just feeling spread too thin. It actually has many negative health effects on the body. It has been estimated that women who experience high levels of stress are 40 percent more likely to experience a stroke or heart attack. Unfortunately, heart disease is the number one cause of death for women in the United States. As if heart disease wasn't scary enough, there are other numerous health problems that result from stress.

- Significant psychological and emotional stress causes imbalances in the body that can lead to hair loss.

- Prolonged amounts of stress can also lead to increases in stomach acid causing discomfort, indigestion, or even IBS and ulcers.

- Additionally, a stressed body often has hormone imbalances, which can lead to irregularities with periods.

- Extreme stress often triggers depression which can worsen the problems for women. • Along with stress comes elevated levels of cortisol, which has shown to decrease and suppress the body's natural sex hormones, leading to decreased sex drive.

- Side effects of changing hormones include acne breakouts, weight gain and insomnia.

As you can see, stress unfortunately effects every part of a woman's body. For these reasons, and the overall wellbeing for women out there, understanding and managing stress is crucial to survival and enjoyment of life.

2. The Stress Response

What is Stress Exactly?

When a person encounters something stressful, the brain sends a signal to the adrenal glands to release various hormones such as noradrenaline, adrenaline and cortisol. These hormones race through the body to prepare the body to flight or fight. The lungs take in more oxygen as the breath quickens. Fats and glucose are released into the body to supply for energy needs during the threat. The senses sharpen to make the body more aware and alert. The heart starts to beat faster, sometimes up to five times faster than normal. As the heart pounds faster, blood pressure rises and certain blood vessels constrict to direct blood flow to the muscles and brain. The muscles in the body tighten enabling the body to act if needed.

In essence, you feel like you got an electric shock. You are prepared to run for your life from a bear, except that you are more likely dealing with an issue at work which requires some creative problem solving. Or perhaps, you are at home after a long day at the office, burnt dinner and have a hungry family staring at you. You don't need to fight or run from anything, not yet anyway, you just need to come up with another solution to feed your family. Unfortunately for women, stress doesn't make problem solving easier. Our emotional response can cause us to become overwhelmed and shut down.

Stress and the Effects on the Male vs. Female Brain

Strangely enough, men and women respond to stress in different ways. The difference in reactions between the genders can impact job performance. For example, researchers at University of Pennsylvania School of Medicine conducted an experiment in how this stress response varies by gender. An even amount of men and women were given a complex math problem and the researcher's cortisol levels, heart rate, perceived stress levels and cerebral blood flow.
In this study, men responded to stress differently than women. Men responded by an increase in cerebral blood flow in the right

prefrontal cortex, which the area of the brain responsible for problem is solving. In women, the area activated was the limbic system. This is the area most responsible for emotion. The researchers also discovered that stress lasted longer in women than men. It is believed that these discoveries are opening the door to discovering why women tend to be more susceptible to stress and anxiety.

Men are primarily strategic thinkers. When it comes to making decisions, they are likely to make a decision based on how likely they are to lose or win in a situation. Sometimes, they start to doubt if they can handle the task. If they decide they can handle the risk, the men go for it. If they decide that they probably can't handle the risk, they tend to avoid or procrastinate.

With men, it is thought that doubt is influenced by knowledge and personal confidence. For example, a senior executive will have more real-world understanding and knowledge of his capabilities. Because of this, he will either use his skills for deeper repertoire to win or choose to fight, or he will strategically withdraw. A worker, on the other hand, with lesser skills may want to hide, delay or withdraw when faced with possible failure. However, his enthusiasm for the new skill may send him rushing into a losing situation. But, that is how men tend to learn.

While there can be exceptions when it comes to responding to stress when dealing with assessment of a situation, the process that men take is typically the same; stress begins when the man receives the assignment, he starts to doubt himself, and the outcome depends on if he decides to act or not.

In comparison, women tend to generally think more communally. Women master the art of relationships. They value the safety and security of the "tribe" and prefer a community, which can be very effective in a work environment. Because of this, when stressful situations arise, they tend to go the opposite route from men. They are less likely to go-it-alone and instead respond by befriending. They aim to build community, while talking with friends, family and co-workers. They seek advice and build the structures that security and safety depend on. While there may always be exceptions to this rule, there is a universal structure in the response. Women do also of course have the ability to go through stressful situations on their own; and have shown a tendency to do so in work environments. This is the dual nature of women's logic.

Balancing the Masculine and Feminine

Many women have started to tap into their masculine energy to be successful in the corporate workplace. However, when it comes to being fulfilled in matters of the heart and home, there can be a problem. While I managed a large team of employees and was head of a team of leaders all day, I would come home and need to be vulnerable, kind and understanding to the needs and requests of my husband. It was a difficult transition at times.

What has granted a woman success in the workplace, does not work in a relationship with a masculine man. In fact, many powerful, successful women are single and do not understand why. This is often because the same energy that has rewarded them at work, typically does not reward them in their role at home. There needs to be a slight adjustment for women to be successful in both areas.

Often, it is a challenge for women to remember that being feminine does not mean being weak. The intuition, flow and beauty are necessary parts of any woman's life, and it is the most useful in home and in our relationships. Balancing the two energies is the challenge of the modern day woman.
Challenges and obstacles will be present that is clear. However, by finding techniques and strategies to manage stress and find a balance, women can reach their optimal level of success in their career and home life. Let's start by taking a look at the different sources of stress that come about both in the workplace and at home.

3. Sources of Stress

In the Workplace

Stress from Upper Management

In the fast paced work environment that most corporate companies are accustomed to, stress is passed along like in a game of dominos. When there is a problem at the top, it is sent down all the way to the bottom. This can present a stressor, as immediate actions may be demanded. Additionally, expectations within the workplace are becoming more demanding- quotas are higher, deadlines are faster. When a goal seems unrealistic, and you have a team to get buy in from, this creates stress. This is even further exasperated when your livelihood depends on reaching that goal.

Gender Inequality

Women often feel less appreciated than men when it comes to opportunities for promotions and compensation. For example, the healthcare industry is largely female-based. It is estimated that 80 percent of workers are female. However, men are still earning more in healthcare careers. Female doctors, on average, earn less than their male counterparts. Male nurses are estimated to earn more than female nurses at every level of education.

Healthcare isn't the only workplace still lacking gender equality. According to a recent survey, male authors were often featured three to four times more than their female counterparts in literary publications such as Harpers Magazine and The New York Review of Books.

Lack of Respect

Even when women do conquer the corporate ladder and land a high level position, there is still the struggle of gaining respect from peers. Some men may have problems with women in power.

Women typically have to work harder to gain respect and be taken seriously among their peers. This added element of being a woman in the workplace only adds stress to a job.

Faster Speed of Business with Advanced Technology

Our bodies are hard wired with the same flight or fight response to stress that we have always had. However, our sources of stress have changed from our previous ancestors, but our subconscious perceives these threats as a life and death confrontation. Even if the change can potentially be positive, our body responds with flight or fight and emotions. Many stressors today are mental, and received via email, text or meeting. They are not immediate threats to our bodies, but still feel that way. With businesses utilizing technology, the speed of transactions if faster than ever before, so stressors are also presented much more frequently.

Long hours in the work place have led to back strain, eye strain, neck problems, wrist problems and increased body weight. Humans are used to evolution that would have taken thousands of years to develop. However, in today's world, the accelerated pace of change has a tendency to overwhelm the majority of people. New strategies and tactics are needed to handle the many stressors that come about to avoid a rollercoaster of cortisol.

What do the Stats Say?

As we discussed earlier, women are no strangers to being in male-dominated work environment. Women typically make up a small amount of officers on corporate boards. In 2012, it was estimated that women held just over 10 percent of these corporate seats around the globe. Other studies of women who haven't quite made it to corporate level, have revealed the challenges they still face to get to the top.

In this survey, up to 87 percent of female board directors have reported needing to overcome obstacles related to gender. About 20 percent have said they aren't listened to and aren't considered an equal or part of the "in" crowd. They also said they have troubles establishing credibility amongst their peers. Five percent said they faced stereotypes of expected female behavior.

On the other hand, when men were polled about these types of challenges in the workplace, 56 percent of men said that females do not face any challenges that are different than men. Of those who admitted to women having faced challenges, more than a quarter blamed these problems on lack of industry knowledge or experience as the problem. Only 22 percent blamed any gender inequality on prejudice or bias and 14 percent thought that women must work harder to prove themselves.

The survey also discovered that women might need to work harder to be positioned in boards.
But once on these boards, the women were often appointed to lead roles such as president or CEO. The researchers noted that in order to receive invitations to boards, women might need to be more accomplished then men.

Women also need to take personal sacrifices to get top positions in the corporate world. In the study, fewer of these women were married or had children compared to their male counterparts; and a larger amount were divorced. These trends tended to be stronger in the United States as opposed to other developed countries. The study found that a greater percentage of female directors outside the United States had children and were married. This may be due to the lack of paid leave and childcare available to those in the U.S.

In fact, in the United States, women only hold 16.6 percent of board seats. On the other hand, Norway has a quota requiring companies to have at least 40 percent of women in board seats. Finland and Sweden are just under 30 percent in this regard.

Companies may have a lot to gain by putting more women in the position of power. A study found that companies with diverse gender boards outperformed male-only boards by 26 percent. Another study discovered that boards with at least three directors with both genders had a larger return on equity and net profit margin.

In the Home

Now let's look at the stress factors common in the home life of a woman.

The Perfect Wife, Mother and Daughter Expectations

Women are social and expected to be caretakers of others. Sociologists have described women as struggling to achieve the "male standard" at work, while also struggling to maintain the status of perfect wife and mother at home. The perfect wife and mother in modern times is still expected to provide her family with home cooked meals, a clean home, care for her husband's needs and don't forget being a soccer mom. Nowadays meals are expected to be organic, Non-GMO and non-processed, clothes are expected to be hand-sewn and special events are expected to look like a designer magazine layout off Pinterest. Women have many pressures and expectations put on them, which are difficult to meet with a full time job.

Women also find it harder to say no to others' requests and have guilty feelings if they can't please everyone. When this happens, women tend to neglect nurturing their own physical and emotional needs because it is perceived as being selfish. This leads to burn out and self-neglect.

Family Specific Mental Labor

A recent study found that while both men and women think about family throughout the day, only women are prone to stress and anxiety produced from family matters. When mothers engage in this family-specific mental labor, it negatively affected their well-being. Some people believe this is because mothers take the role of household managers which leads them to think about the more unpleasant aspects of family care.

I know I have experienced this first-hand. It goes something like this: thinking about a problem your child is having at school with a friend and how to talk to them about it, thinking about an upcoming holiday you have to plan for, pondering how the water heater broke and that you need to budget some money to fix it and wondering what you are going to do about your dog that chewed up your new couch leg.

Finding Balance

Two of the most important aspects in women's lives are work and family. Balancing these two aspects is becoming a key issue in many societies. There are many facets in a woman's life that can subject her to stress. An imbalance in work and family life can arise due to a variety of factors, and these factors can strengthen the brunt of pressure on women.

Traditionally, the major responsibility of women has been the maintenance of family that includes home and childcare. Breadwinning was left to be the major responsibility of men. But with more women pursuing careers and entering the workforce, these gender roles are changing, and men are often not taking on the roles at home.

Unfortunately, stress that affects a woman's work life can be carried over into the home. Job instability, role overload and inadequate childcare can be stressful. In order for women to balance this stress, she needs to know that her career is important and she is not sacrificing their child's wellbeing in order to benefit themselves. Often, mothers can feel like they are abandoning their child to other caregivers. It is difficult to find the balance and this is often a daily struggle for many women.

4. Learn and Recognize the Signs of Stress

Many times, people are stressed and do not even know it. The signs of stress can be hard to pinpoint if they are experienced frequently. However, it is imperative to recognize that they are not baseline and are unhealthy. There are different aspects of yourself and your functioning to consider including your cognitive, emotional, physical and behavioral health.

Different Types of Stress Symptoms

Unfortunately, stress affects almost every part of our body. Below we will take a look at the 4 different ways stress is expressed.

Cognitively

Stress will take a toll on mental capacity and debilitate a person. Some cognitive signs include memory problems, poor judgment, focusing on the negative and constant worrying. If you have a hard time concentrating and if you experience anxious, racing thoughts, this is a sign of stress and can be relieved by taking the proper steps.

Emotionally

When a person is stressed, there is a little chance of them being in a good mood. It is chemically improbable. Emotional symptoms of stress show as moodiness and feeling overwhelmed. Those experiencing emotional stress also often have depression and experience general unhappiness. Agitation, inability to relax, a sense of loneliness and isolation are other symptoms of emotional stress.

Physically

Those with chronic stress often exhibit physical symptoms as well. These include aches, pains, nausea and dizziness. Other common symptoms are frequent colds, diarrhea, constipation, chest pain and loss of sex drive.

Behaviorally

Lastly, stress can be exhibited in behavioral symptoms. Sleeping too much or too little is one common sign of stress. Eating more or less is another. Those with chronic stress also tend to neglect and procrastinate with their responsibilities, use drugs or alcohol to relax and establish other nervous habits.

While these are all common signs of stress, keep in mind that other psychological or medical problems could be causing these symptoms as well. If you are experiencing symptoms, you may want to consider seeing a doctor for a full evaluation. All of these symptoms are detrimental to success at home or at work.

5. Techniques for Confronting and Managing Stress

We know the main reasons that women are stressed in modern times, and what that stress does to the body. Now let's look at what you can do to face stress head on and take control of the triggers. With understanding and effort, it is possible to overcome the stress you experience and achieve the life you want.

I faced my own battles against stress between work and home, and have compiled these techniques which I have found most effective. The stress triggers have not gone away, but my reaction to them has changed. This, you will learn, makes all the difference. Not all of these will work for everyone, but experimenting with different strategies will allow you to find which ones works best for you.

Strengthen Emotional Intelligence

Out of all the skills that are essential in the workplace, emotional intelligence is at the top of the list for women. This is the ability to recognize, assess and control emotions. Women are wired to experience powerful feelings and emotions, which can overpower us if we are not aware of how they work. They can alternatively be important and helpful signs. However, when stress hits, it is harder to handle emotions and they even impact the ability to listen effectively and make decisions. Here are the basics to developing emotional intelligence, so that when stressors do come, you can be prepared.

Attributes of Emotional Intelligence

There are four key attributes of emotional intelligence: self-awareness, self-management, social awareness and relationship management.

Self-awareness is the ability to recognize your own emotions and how they affect behavior and thoughts. It will also allow you to have self-confidence along with knowing your strengths and weaknesses.

Self-management allows you to control behaviors and impulsive feelings. It also allows you to take initiative, manage emotions in healthy ways, adapt to circumstances and follow through with commitments to others.

Social awareness is elemental to emotional intelligence because it allows you to understand the needs, emotions and concerns of others. When you have social awareness, you can also pick up more on emotional cues, which allow you to feel comfortable in social situations and see the power of dynamics while in a group.

Relationship management is also an important element of emotional intelligence. If you have this, you will be able to inspire and influence others, manage conflict, work well on a team and communicate clearly.

5 Key Skills Required

Reducing stress also helps to build emotional intelligence. When your emotional intelligence is developed, you will also be able to remain focused and stay connected to others. This is accomplished by learning key skills. Here are five of those skills in further detail: The ability to reduce stress in a variety of situations. Building emotional intelligence is part of learning to control oneself. When you have the power to reduce the stress in any situation, you are taking charge and building emotional intelligence.

The ability to recognize certain emotions and stop them from making you feel overwhelmed. When you have emotional intelligence, you can recognize that certain emotions can be toxic to your mind and body. If you have the ability to stop them, you remain in control of your body and are less likely to be overwhelmed.

The ability to connect with others using nonverbal communication. Emotional intelligence grants you the power to read others' emotions without words being spoken. When you can do so, you are a better communicator and have greater understanding.

The ability to use play and humor to connect in stressful situations. If you are in a stressful situation, and other people are involved, it shows great emotional intelligence to try to diffuse the situation with humor or play. Being able to successfully diffuse a situation with these tools displays great emotional intelligence.

The ability to resolve conflicts with confidence. Those with emotional intelligence have the ability to resolve conflicts on a positive note. They also can handle these stressful situations with confidence. This is a key competency for leaders and managers in the workplace.

Understand How to Build a Stress Tolerance

In order to survive in a high-stress environment, you will have to evaluate how much stress you can handle. Different people can handle different amounts, and it will vary from person to person. Some people are able to handle a larger amount of stress and can even thrive in that type of environment. While others will need to pace themselves. The ability to tolerate stress will depend on certain factors like your general outlook on life, the quality of relationships you have, genetics and emotional intelligence.

In order to increase your stress tolerance level, take the following steps:

1. Build a strong, supportive network. Building a strong network of supportive family and friends can be a huge buffer in the fight against life's stresses. Keep in mind that the more isolated and lonely you are, the more prone you are to stress.

2. To tackle stress, improve your sense of control. It is often easier to handle stress if you have confidence in your ability to persevere through challenges and events that cause stress. When you feel in control, you are less likely to experience more stress symptoms.

3.	Another important element to tackling stress is to change your outlook and attitude. It has been shown that optimistic people tend to handle stress better than their pessimistic peers. Try to embrace challenges with a strong sense of humor and accept change as a part of your life.

4.	Try to take charge of your emotions. Studies have shown that those who do not know how to calm or soothe themselves, are more prone to stress. If you are feeling sad or overwhelmed at a situation, having the ability to balance your emotions will keep stress away.

5.	Prepare yourself for being stressed. The more information you have about a stressful situation, the more you will find it easier to cope. Painting a realistic expectation of the outcome will help you handle any emotional changes and stress.

By practicing these steps, you can increase the amount of stress you can handle each day.
Prioritize
Many women struggle with prioritizing because they feel like everything and everyone is important. I definitely experienced that. However, with focus and effort, I was able to clear up my priorities.

Here are tips I have found helpful:

    a.	Write everything down
When you first wake up and the thoughts of what you need to get done are overwhelming, start by making a list. Write down all the things that need to get done. Once you have the list down, separate items into urgent vs. non-urgent. The urgent priorities are what you have to get done that day.

    b.	Assess value
When certain tasks are completed, they will offer more benefit than others. Outline your priorities into those tasks that have the most value and get them done first.

    c.	Be honest and realistic

Know your limits and try not to set any goals past those limits. Setting goals that are unattainable will only cause disappointment down the road.

  d. Allow for flexibility

All of us know that sometimes, our days do not go according to plan. To effectively prioritize, it is important to be able to deal with changing priorities. Decide if they are urgent and take them as they come.

  e. Let it go

When there is an important priority, it is too easy to get caught up in minor details of the task and end up spending too much time on one task. Doing so will keep you from getting other stuff done. It is important to acknowledge and recognize when this is happening and set deadlines to stop yourself.

By practicing this simple process, you can begin to get the most valuable tasks done each day.

Ask for help

Many women are ashamed or intimidated to ask for help. However, there should be no shame in asking if you can't handle a situation or don't know how to handle it. Too often, asking for help is seen as a sign of being weak of vulnerable, but it can be empowering. The most successful entrepreneurs understand the power of delegation and hiring others who are smarter to them to build the best team possible. A lot of stress, personal burden and time can be saved if you open yourself to help.

  1. Delegation

Delegation is a task that can be difficult for many mothers. We are used to running the show by ourselves and don't even know where to start when it comes to other people helping us. But delegating help is a skill that is important to being successful and healthy. Start by deciding that delegation is a priority and that you are going to do what is necessary to stay sane. To get start delegating, start with these steps.

a.   What? First, admit to yourself that you can't do everything that needs to be done and stop adding things to your list. Make the decision that you are going to seek help. Start by thinking about an area of your life that is stressful and you dread doing. Perhaps this is the area to ask for help.

b.   Who? Finding someone to take care of things for you may seem impossible. It's not enough to say that you're going to ask someone to help you, but the hardest part is probably finding who. You're going to need to find someone who you are comfortable in giving even your toughest tasks. It may take a bit of effort at first, but once you have an established list of people you can rely on, it can be comforting and relaxing.

First, start by going through friends and family. Can any of them help you with what you need to get done? If not, ask friends and family who could help you. See if any of them can recommend professionals who offer the service you are looking for. Chances are there is someone out there who is more than willing to help if you just ask.

c.   How? When you have found someone to help you, be specific as possible. If you would like something done a certain way, then make sure to let that person know. Try to be as clear as possible with what you want done and how you'd like it to be done.

Additional Tips

Once you have decided to delegate a task, then try to trust that person to get the job done. Don't waste the time and the energy thinking about them getting the job done. When they are finished, it is time to check and ensure the job was done properly. If it was great, mission accomplished. If not, coach them for next time and evaluate if they are likely to get it right in the future. Eventually you will learn to find those you can trust and better ways to communicate your needs as well.

Develop Positive Habits

One of the biggest wastes of time is complaining. If you want to tackle stress, then stop complaining. It doesn't help anyone, especially you. It may feel good to vent every now and then, but venting really doesn't get you anywhere. If you are upset and want to something to change, then take positive action. Start by asking yourself how you can solve a problem and what you can do to resolve a situation. Steer clear from negative people that give you unnecessary anxiety and worry. Try to smile more. You may have to force if at first, but the more you smile and laugh, the happier you will be. When you are happy, you are more likely to attract positive situations into your life. Have a clean heart that holds no grudges, ill-will, envy or anger towards anyone. It is only negative energy that will get you down. If you can help it, don't allow every little thing to ruin your mood. Focus on improving communication, self-development and relationships.

Examples of positive habits to work on

a.   Be grateful. Make it a habit of being thankful for what you have and focus on the good things in your life. It is too easy to get in the habit of worrying over little things that get in the way of appreciating what is important like friends, family, freedom, good health and other opportunities that we enjoy. Getting caught up in little details undermines the fact that we really do have a lot to be grateful for.

b.   Practice being a good listener. You will find that others have a lot to say if you're willing to listen. Take the time to listen to others' points of view. You may not agree with what they have to say, but put yourself in their place and try to understand where they are coming from.

c.   Purposefully perform an act of kindness. Do something nice for someone else just for the sake of doing an act of service. Try helping an elderly person with their groceries or with their mail. Offer to tend your friend's children or do another element of service that is not in your routine. Doing a small, simple act of service will make you feel better and promotes a feeling of good will.

d.   Tell friends and family you appreciate them. Our loved ones like to hear how much they mean to us. It is often our closest family and friends that we take for granted. If you take the time to tell someone else how much you appreciate them, it will make you and your loved one feel good.

e.   Have a good laugh. Try telling a joke or reading the comics to help loosen up. Make plans to see a new comedy movie that you've wanted to see for a while. Laughter and lightheartedness relieve stress and change your outlook on life. If you want to stay on top of your mood, plan on doing things to make yourself happy every day.

f.   Smile at someone. This is probably the easiest thing you can do today. If you pass someone on the street or in the hall, take the time to make eye contact and smile. Say hi and acknowledge them. Doing this will make you feel good and make the other person feel good. Typically, we are so wrapped up in our own lives that we don't notice people around us.

g.   Be determined to hold a positive mindset. When you wake up in the morning, make the commitment to face the day with a positive attitude. Acknowledge that there are probably a few things that won't go your way or as smoothly as you planned, but be willing to tackle these challenges that come your way with a positive attitude.

Create a Work Life Balance

The long hours that you put in at work may make you feel like work is your only priority. After all, it is work that helps to pay for your shelter and food to survive. But more important than work are the relationships with your loved ones. It is important to create a balance between different aspects of your life such as health, finance, spiritual and personal relationships. All of these elements of your life are just as important as work, and it is important to balance them for a healthy life. Take the time to examine your daily life. Are you finding any elements that are lopsided? Are you spending too much time in one area of your life as opposed to the other? Take note as to what you can do to balance these elements in your life.

1. Balance achievement and enjoyment

In trying to find balance, keep in mind that balance will not mean spending equal amounts of time between all the elements in your life. It is not realistic. Life should be more fluid than that. Also, the right balance for you today may not be the right balance tomorrow. The truth is that there is no perfect, one-size balance that you should be striving for. As you live your life with work and home life, you will eventually find the balance that you need and that works for you.

2. Four quadrants of home and work

It is possible to have meaningful enjoyment and balance between the four quadrants. These quadrants are family, friends, work and self. To find balance in your life, start by asking yourself when the last time you achieved and enjoyed something at work. When was the last time you achieved and enjoyed something with family and friends? When was the last time you enjoyed and achieved something for you?

Try spending a short amount of quality time doing something you enjoy. When you get home from work, decide if you are going to spend the night enjoying or achieving.

When you get home, act accordingly. When you are at work, make sure you are achieving but also enjoying that sense of achievement.

3. Tips

Many people find that they feel balanced when achievement and enjoyment are balanced. Head to work with an optimistic point of view that you are going to achieve a lot and that you are going to enjoy the achievement. If no one else pats you on the back for an achievement, then take the time to do it for yourself. Help and lift others along the way. Making the environment around you positive reaps benefits for you and others. Others will be drawn to you when you are positive and kind.

These simple concepts, when applied, will make a big difference in your day. If you focus on these key components of your day, you will see big changes. Make it a point to make these habits a part of your daily routine for the rest of your life.

Eat a Healthy Diet

There's always the saying that you are what you eat. If you are choosing to fuel your body with unhealthy food, you are going to be unhealthy. Add stress to this type of environment, and you are headed for a train wreck. Eating healthy is of the utmost importance when it comes to tackling stress and taking care of yourself. I found I had a renewed energy, and slimmer waist line, when I made healthy eating a priority.

Here are some tips:

Food can reduce stress levels
Healthy food is one of the simplest ways to relieve stress. Foods that contain high vitamins and minerals help to refuel the body and reduce stress.

    a.   Foods to include

When you are taking care of your body, make sure to drink a lot of water. Eat plenty of fresh fruits and vegetables. For healthy proteins, eat fish and yogurt. Soups are often full of vegetables and can help you feel full at dinnertime. Herbal products often contain plenty of vitamins and minerals that can help your body recover from large amounts of stress.

    b.   Foods to avoid

It is important to take note that certain foods can aggravate stress. While you do not have to avoid these foods completely, strive to eat them only in moderation. Coffee, tea, energy drinks and cocoa can increase stress in the body. Fast food and other processed food are often not healthy and have minimal amounts of nutrition for the body, which can also trigger the stress response. Limit the amount of butter, cheese, sugar, alcohol, meat and shellfish that is consumed in your diet as well. Other foods that can trigger and aggravate stress are coconut oil, almonds and other types of nuts.

Calm Your Mind

Worrying is a waste of time and energy, just like complaining. It also adds to a stressful situation and doesn't help things get better. To calm your mind, try to accept things you can't change and avoid dwelling on the past.

Techniques

Women with increased levels of nervous tension and anxiety can benefit from the following calming techniques. Often times many women have trouble quieting their mind and have to sift through a steady stream of negative "self-talk." As the day goes by, the mind may be flooded with fantasies, feelings and thoughts that cause emotional responses. These thoughts often focus on unresolved issues from work, personal relationships, finances and health. The replay of these issues can be exhausting and reinforce anxiety symptoms. To tackle the challenge of quieting your mind, try some of these techniques.

a.   Focus. Start by selecting a personal object that you care for. Focus your attention and energy on this object for few minutes who you inhale and exhale. Try not to let any other thoughts or feelings enter the mind during this exercise. If thoughts come into the mind, just return them to the object. At the end of the exercise, you may find yourself being calmer and more peaceful. Any tension that existed at the beginning of the exercise should be diminished.

b.   Meditation. To do this exercise, lie or sit in a comfortable position. Breathe deeply and close your eyes. Breathe relaxed and slow. Focus your attention on breathing and take note of the movement of your chest moving in and out. Block out other thoughts, sensations and feelings. If your attention wanders, return the focus to your breathing. On the inhale, say the word "peace" and on the exhale, say the word "calm." When you repeat these words, you will be able to concentrate. Continue this practice until you feel relaxed.

c. Grounding. Women who suffer from anxiety can feel disorganized and ungrounded. It is a sense of "falling apart." When an anxiety episode hits, it can take a concentrated effort just to get through the day. Grounding techniques can help you feel more focused and centered. When these techniques are practiced, your energies will be organized and you'll have the energy to proceed with your day.

The first grounding technique is the oak tree meditation. Start by sitting in a comfortable position with arms resting at sides. Breathe deeply and close your eyes. Keep breathing relaxed and slow. Imagine that your body is a strong oak tree. Imagine that your body is the strong trunk and the roots are your legs, stretching deep into the earth. When stress comes your way, imagine that you are deeply rooted and cannot be shaken easily. It will help you keep calm, confident and relaxed.

Another grounding technique is the grounding cord meditation. To do this, sit in a comfortable position with arms resting at the sides. Close your eyes and breathe deeply. Let the breathing be relaxed and slow. Try to imagine a wide, thick cord attached to the base of your spine. This cord helps to ground you. Imagine that this cord hooks itself inside the earth into solid bedrock. Keep breathing deeply. If stress comes your way, imagine that this cord is binding you to the earth.

d. Discovering/Releasing Muscle Tension. One of the most unpleasant side effects of stress is muscle tension. It can be debilitating and painful. To help relieve tension, practice these exercises.

First, you must start by discovering the muscle tension. Lie on your back comfortably. Allow the arms to rest at the sides with palms down. Raise your right hand and hold it elevated for 15 seconds. Try to take note if your forearm is tense or tight. Drop your arm down and relax. Repeat this with your left arm. If you are laying still, you may notice that other parts of the body are sore and tight. Once you have identified what muscles need help, then move on to relieve the muscles.

      e. Shrinking stress

Start by laying on your back comfortably resting arms at the sides. Slowly breathe in and out. Clench fists and hold them tightly for about 15 seconds. While you are clenching your fists, relax the rest of the body. Imagine the fists becoming tighter and tighter. Then slowly let the hands relax. While you are allowing the hands to relax, imagine a glowing light flowing through your body. This light makes your muscles pliable and soft. Then, tense and relax the your body starting from the face, then moving to the shoulders, then back, then stomach, moving to the pelvis, then legs, then the feet and toes. Hold each body part tense for 15 seconds then relax for 30 seconds before moving to other body parts. Finish by shaking out hands and imagine tension moving out of the fingertips.

    f.   Erasing stress

Another tension relieving exercise starts in the same position as the previous exercise. While you are laying on the floor, be aware of tight and knotted parts of the body. Take note of how they feel. Do you also feel other strong feelings such as anger or pain in these parts of the body? While you are breathing, release these anxious feelings with your breath, lowering these feelings until they fade.

Get Enough Sleep

Some days, it may seem impossible to get enough sleep with your busy schedule. But it is important to get at least 6-8 hours of sleep each night to help keep your stress levels in check.

How stress and sleep relate

Sadly, most people don't get enough sleep. It is estimated that three out of four don't. This may be because stress and sleep are closely related. When our body is constantly flooded with stress hormones, it may be nearly impossible to relax and go to sleep. When the stress response is constantly triggered in the body and isn't resolved through relaxation, you can end up with chronic stress. This happens when your body is constantly stressed and doesn't have the opportunity to rest and recover.

How much sleep do you need?

Sleep requirements vary by age and lifestyle requirements. While there are "rule-of-thumb" amounts of sleep that experts have agreed on, it is important to note your own individual needs by determining how you feel on different amounts of sleep.

There is no magic number of sleep partly because the amount of sleep you require on a daily basis is based on two different factors on people's sleep. For example, a person's basal sleep requirement is the amount of sleep we need on a regular basis for the best performance. Sleep debt is the amount of accumulated sleep that we lose to poor sleep habits. Studies have suggested that healthy adults need about seven to eight hours of sleep every night, but the interaction between basal sleep and sleep debt can make things complicated. For instance, you may be sleeping enough at night but still have unresolved sleep debt that can make you feel sleepy or less alert at times.

Some good news, however, is that researchers believe that unresolved sleep can be "paid off." Although there are still ongoing studies related to basal and unresolved sleep, it is well known that lack of sleep in general causes serious health consequences that can jeopardize your safety.
Try keeping a log of your sleep and how you feel with different amounts of sleep. Aim for at least seven to eight hours a night for a starting point.

How to Improve Sleep

If you want to improve your sleeping habits, here are a few suggestions to try. Along with testing various amounts of sleep and keeping a log, keep assessing your habits. Pay attention to your mood, health and energy. In addition, there are a variety of things to help you get more shut-eye at night.

- To start, establish consistent sleep and wake routines, even on weekends.

- Create a regular bedtime routine that helps you relax, such as listening to soothing music or soaking in a hot bath.

- Start your bedtime routine about an hour before you expect to fall asleep.

- Make your sleep environment as comfortable as possible. Try to make it quiet, dark and cool.

- Sleep on pillows and a comfortable mattress.

- Keep distractions out of the bedroom such as TVs, computers and avoid reading in bed.

- Finish eating two to three hours before your bedtime as well.

- Having a consistent exercise schedule will help you fall asleep better, but do not work out close to bedtime hours.

- Above all, make sleep a priority. Don't put it off until everything else is done. Stop doing tasks and chores at your established bedtime so you can get some good, quality sleep.

Enjoy the Outdoors

This may be a low priority on your list, but it can make a big difference in how you feel throughout the day. Make it a goal to at least take a walk outside every day. A walk surrounded by nature and fresh air can help relieve stress.

Health benefits of being outside
There is one immediate health benefit that we reap from being outside and that is absorption of Vitamin D. We are constantly learning more about Vitamin D, including how good it is for our health. It helps to prevent cancer, obesity, inflammation and hormonal problems. It improves our immune system. Because sunlight is one of the only sources of Vitamin D, it makes sense to get outside as much as possible.

Getting outside helps to improve sleep as well. Studies have shown that natural sunlight helps to set the body's internal clock that normalizes functions to tell us when to sleep and eat. As we have discussed above, sleep is critical to our overall health.

Getting outside also gives us a break from technology and other fast-paced stresses of the world. We tend to have a clearer, more focused mind when we are outside. Some others take this time of being outside to enjoy and learn a new skill or physical activity.

Being out in nature has been proven to calm our bodies and minds. It helps to lower our stress levels and blood pressure. In Japan, there are Forest Therapy trails that encourage people to get outside and receive nature therapy.

Nature helps to soothe our senses. Studies have shown that many people find that bird songs help to calm and reassure people. The smell of crisp, clean air is also closely linked to parts of our brain responsible for processing emotion. Scents that we inhale have an immediate impact in our body. Plants have been shown to emit phytoncides which are organic compounds along with essential oil. When we inhale these phytoncides, we reduce anxiety and slow down breathing.

Ideas to Get Outdoors

If going for walks outside sounds boring and unappealing to you, then don't fret. There are other ways to spend time outside that may piqué your interest. Gardening is one that will reap benefit too. From planting flowers, to vegetable garden, gardening gets you outside and communing with nature regularly.

Try taking vacations in beautiful places. This doesn't mean that you have to do extensive traveling, either. There are beautiful places all around. Visit a local state or national park. Pack up and head to a nearby beach. Look for landscapes that make you interested in getting outside.

Look for local trails for hiking and biking. Chances are, there are plenty of trails near you that are pretty and will allow you to get some fresh air. Another suggestion is to simply try sitting outside. In our culture, we are constantly on the go. If you need a break, try sitting outside and simply appreciating the natural beauty around you. Focus on discovering new sights, scents and sounds while you focus on the moment. Find a local park for an outdoor workout. If you're not sure what park is the best, ask around.

Lastly, make it a point to commit to the outdoors. Whether there it is rainy or sunny, you can enjoy the outdoors in a variety of temperatures if you are covered up properly. Starting with at least 30 minutes a day will work positive benefits into your life.

Connect with Loved Ones

Spending time with loved ones decreases stress and plants joy in the heart.

Social connections and happiness

While we may live in an individualistic society, it has been proven that we all need people around us to thrive and be happy. We need close relationships to function normally and well.
Loving relationships are critical to our happiness because they create safety and psychological space that allows us to explore and learn. When we feel supported and safe, there is no need to focus on feelings of survival. We have more opportunities to explore our world and the opportunity to reduce stress.

One characteristic of a close relationship is the ability to love and be loved. With close relationships, there is a mutual understanding that allows for better communication. There is also caring and a source of direct help in times of trouble. Close relationships give us the validation of self-worth and a sense of security. While you're in a close relationship, you will have the opportunity to celebrate good times and have a diversity of ideas to help us learn and grow. Being in a close relationship can be fun as you can cherish having a close companion.

When we are part of a close-knit community, we have a sense of identity. We are able to understand who we are and have a feeling that we are part of something bigger. Those with strong social connections have fewer stress-related problems, faster recoveries from illness and lower risk of mental illness. People in our close relationships can also support and encourage us to have healthy habits like moderation and exercise.

Studies have also shown that unlike materialistic things, close relationships typically last longer. We aim to want close relationships and receive positive emotions from them.

Schedule time for you
While it is important to spend time with loved ones, it is also important to spend time with ourselves. Giving ourselves solitude is something that is rare these days. We are constantly connected to each other. In fact, our culture seems to equate solitude with those who are sad or lonely. However, seeking solitude can be quite healthy. There are actually quite a few psychological and physical benefits to spending time alone.

Benefits
a.	Improve concentration. When we are constantly surrounded by distractions, we aren't able to concentrate as well. When these distractions are removed, it will give your brain more time to concentrate which allows for more work to be done in a shorter amount of time.

b.	Unwind. When your brain is constantly "on", it doesn't have the opportunity to rest and replenish itself. When you are by yourself with no distractions, you'll have a clear mind and will be able to think more clearly. It gives you the opportunity to revitalize the body and brain at the same time.

c.	Reboot the brain. Seeking solitude allows you to get back to the simple things in life. You have time to unwind and think simple thoughts. It also gives the brain a rest, so it has more energy to tackle things later.

d.   Find your voice. While being a part of a group is important, it is also critical to establish your own thoughts and decisions. Having time to yourself allows you to make your own thoughts and choices.

e.   Learn about yourself. In solitude, you'll have the opportunity to sort out problems and thoughts by yourself. This allows you to figure out how you make choices.

f.   Work through problems. When you are surrounded by distractions and other information, it is hard to think through your own problems. Solitude allows you the time and energy to figure out how you deal with complex issues in your life.

g.   Think deeply. Daily commitments and responsibilities can be overwhelming. When you experience solitude, you can engage in deep thought which inhibits creativity.

Tips

• If it seems hard for you to find solitude, then you may have to schedule it. Make time each day to unplug from the phone and the Internet. If you must use the computer, then turn off any alerts or incoming message beeps. You will be surprised at how much you can get done once you're not distracted.

• Try waking up about thirty minutes earlier. You can use this time to problem solve, meditate, create or produce. It's also helpful if you can get to work before everyone arrives and the phones start ringing.

• Some people find that scheduling the same time every day helps them to get solitude time. Solitude time does not have to be long, but it should be long enough to give you time to focus, meditate, create or think deeply.

6. Conclusion

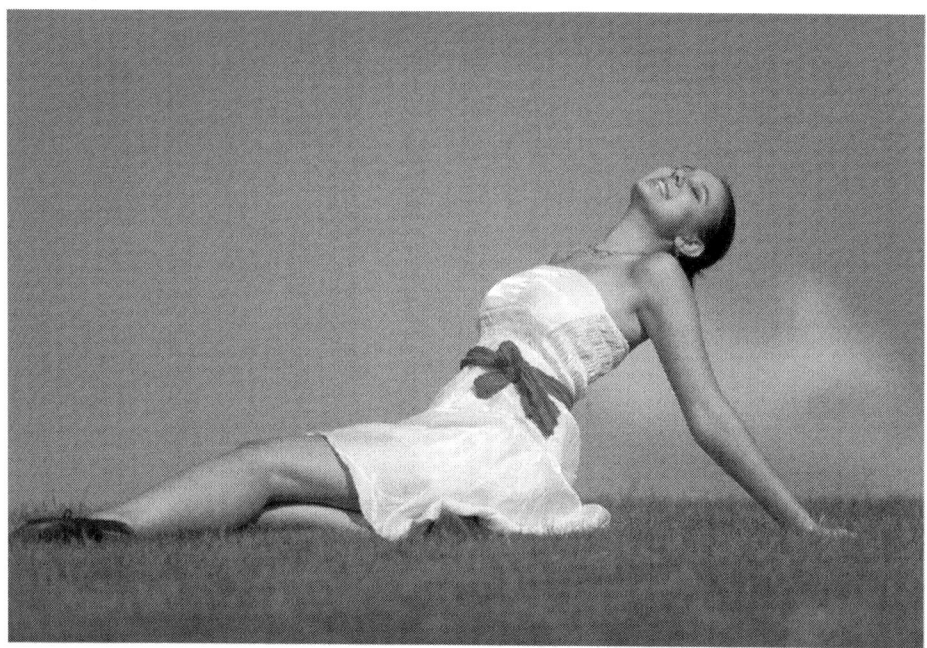

In this book, we have outlined many things can help us, as working mothers, to take control of our lives and reduce stress. It is easy to become a victim to our circumstances and let things take over our lives that we cannot seem to control. But it is important to remember that we do have control of our own lives. Simply put, reducing stress and chaos in our lives start with us.

As we aim to take care of careers and our families, we need to put ourselves first. For many women, including me, this is probably the most difficult part. But work, housework and childcare can't be done if we are sick or feeling terrible. When we take the time to get enough sleep, eat healthy, reduce stress and get time to ourselves, we feel more in control of our lives and can work more effectively.

Each day, remind yourself that you are human and can only do so much. Look at your list and start with the most urgent items. If you do not get everything done on the list, don't be hard on yourself. We are only human, after all. If you had to stay late at work and don't have time to cook dinner, there is no harm in asking your husband to cook or picking up dinner from a restaurant. Do what you need to do to make it through the day.

Above all, remind yourself to enjoy every single day. While each day may go by slowly and sometimes painfully, the years and days go by so fast. Before you know it, these busy years will mostly likely be memories. Stay positive and laugh with your husband and kids. Staying happy and finding these balances in your life will only help you reap benefits in the many years to come.

Printed in Great Britain
by Amazon